Table of Contents

The kidneys are a pair of bean-shaped organs on either side of your spine, below your ribs and behind your belly. Each kidney is about 4 or 5 inches long, roughly the size of a large fist.

The kidneys' job is to filter your blood. They remove wastes, control the body's fluid balance, and keep the right levels of electrolytes. All of the blood in your body passes through them about 40 times a day.

Blood comes into the kidney, waste gets removed, and salt, water, and minerals are adjusted, if needed. The filtered blood goes back into the body. Waste gets turned into urine, which collects in the kidney's pelvis -- a funnel-shaped structure that drains down a tube called the ureter to the bladder.

Each kidney has around a million tiny filters called nephrons. You could have only 10% of your kidneys working, and you may not notice any symptoms or problems.

If blood stops flowing into a kidney, part or all of it could die. That can lead to kidney failure.

BREAKFAST

1. Shakshuka

Prep Time: 10 Minutes

Cook Time: 30 Minutes

Servings: 4

Ingredients

- 3Tbs Olive oil
- 1 red onion, diced
- 1 large red bell pepper, thinly sliced or diced
- 1 large yellow bell pepper, sliced or diced
- 4 garlic cloves, rough chopped
- 3/4 tsp salt, more to taste
- cracked pepper to taste
- 1 tsp cumin
- 1 tsp sugar
- 1 tsp smoked paprika
- 1/2 tsp aleppo chili flakes (optional)

- 3 medium tomatoes diced small with juices (or one 14-ounce can diced tomatoes with juices)
- 1/3 cup water or white wine
- 2 tablespoons fresh basil ribbons, chopped cilantro or Italian parsley
- 4 –6 Extra large organic eggs

Other optional additions:

- 1/4 – 1/2 cup goat cheese or crumbled feta
- ¼ C finely diced Spanish-style cured Chorizo or 1 cup Merguez Sausage,

Instructions

1. preheat oven to 375F
2. In a large cast iron skillet, heat the olive oil over medium heat. Add the onion and cook until tender, about 5 minutes. Add the sliced peppers and garlic, and turn heat down to med-low and cook for 5-7 more minutes, until peppers are tender.
3. Add all spices, sugar and salt.
4. Cook for 2 more minutes. Add fresh tomatoes and water (or wine).

5. Simmer on low for 10-15 minutes, uncovered, adding more water if it gets too dry or thick. You want a saucy, stew-like consistency. After tomatoes cook down, taste, it should be full-flavored, so adjust salt, spices, and sugar if necessary.

6. With the back of a spoon, make a well for each egg in the stew. Crack the eggs into each well, sprinkling each egg with a little salt and cracked pepper and Aleppo chili flakes.

7. Place in the 375F oven.

8. Bake until egg whites are become opaque and are cooked (about 8-10 minutes) and yolks are still soft (or to your desired doneness.)

9. Remove from oven and top with fresh basil (or cilantro or Italian Parsley) and goat cheese.

10. Serve with crusty bread.

Prep Time: 20 Minutes

Cook Time: 10 Minutes

Servings: 4

Ingredients

- 8 oz chorizo (links or ground) browned (or make this or use vegan chorizo)
- ¾ Cup dry polenta or corn meal
- 2 ½ C chicken stock (or veggie stock)
- 1 Cup grated melting cheese (mozzarella, cheddar, jack)
- ¼ C chopped cilantro divided
- ½ tsp smoked paprika
- salt and pepper to taste
- 6 eggs
- hot sauce for garnish
- variations- see below

Instructions

1. Pre-heat oven to 400F.

2. In a cast iron or oven proof 10 inch skillet, brown sausage or chorizo. Set aside.

3. In the same pan, add stock and bring to a boil. Turn heat to med low, whisk in polenta and smoked paprika, whisking vigorously -to prevent clumping. Once whisked well, cover, turn heat to low and let cook 15 minutes, stirring a few times.

4. Add grated cheese, stir to incorporate. Fold in ½ of the chopped cilantro, ½ of the browned chorizo (or sausage). Taste for salt and add if necessary.(If using chicken stock and chorizo, they will naturally be salty, but you may need to adjust- polenta should be flavorful.) Pepper to taste.

5. Place the other half of the chorizo on top of the polenta, in the center. With a spoon, make small wells in the polenta where the eggs will rest, around the outer edges of the skillet, in a circle. Crack the eggs and place them in the wells. Lightly salt and pepper each egg. Place the skillet in the 400F oven and bake until egg whites are white and set and yolks are set, but still soft (or cook until your desired doneness) .

6. I will often broil for just a quick minute. Garnish with hot sauce and remaining cilantro.

7. Note- You could add a bed sautéed spinach, sautéed peppers, sautéed onions, sautéed mushrooms to this dish, by placing atop the polenta and under the eggs. To get the calories down, leave out the chorizo.

Prep Time: 10 Minutes

Cook Time: 40 Minutes

Servings: 4

Ingredients

- 1–2 tablespoons olive oil
- 1/2 onion- diced
- 3 garlic cloves- minced
- 2 medium tomatoes, diced (or sub pico de gallo)
- 1 can rinsed beans (black bean, pinto, cannellini, or heirloom beans) about 1 1/2 cups
- 1 teaspoon cumin
- 1 teaspoon coriander
- 1/2 teaspoon chipotle powder
- 1/2 teaspoon smoked paprika
- 1/2 teaspoon salt
- cracked pepper
- 2 tablespoons water
- Four 6-inch tortillas (I use a corn and flour blend)
- olive oil for brushing

- 4 eggs (1 egg per serving -you can add more if you want)

Optional:

- 1/2 cup crumbled cotija, queso fresco, feta or goat cheese (optional)

Garnishes:

- 1 large avocado-sliced, 2 tablespoons chopped fresh cilantro,lime wedges, sour cream, Hot Sauce,Pico de gallo

Optional Additions:

- bell pepper, kale, zucchini, mushrooms.

Instructions

1. Preheat oven to 400F.
2. In a large pan over medium heat, saute onion in olive oil until tender, about 5 minutes (at this point, if you are adding other veggies, do this now, cooking until tender). Add garlic, sauté for a minute or two. Add 1/2 of the diced tomatoes (saving half for garnish) and beans, spices, salt, and 2 tablespoons water. Let simmer on med-low until tomatoes break down a bit,

about 5 minutes, stirring occasionally, keeping them nice and warm. Taste and adjust spices and salt to taste.

3. Brush cast-iron skillets (or one large skillet) with olive oil, coating the edges too. Lay tortillas down and brush tops of tortillas with a little olive oil.

4. Divide the warm bean mixture, making little indentations with the back of a spoon, for the eggs to rest in, so they stay in place. (If using a large skillet, layer the tortillas so they come up the sides of the skillet a bit -you may need a couple extra), and spread all of the beans evenly over the tortillas, making indentations for the eggs).

5. Carefully break the eggs and place them in the indentations. Sprinkle eggs with salt and pepper, and if you want, crumbled cheese, and place in the hot oven to bake.

6. Check after 10-12 minutes. Continue cooking until egg whites are white and yolks are to your desired doneness (another 5-10 minutes). Baking will go faster depending on how hot the beans are.

7. Serve with avocado, lime, sour cream, cilantro, hot sauce, and fresh tomatoes.

Prep Time: 35 Minutes

Cook Time: 60 Minutes

Servings: 8-10

Ingredients

- 16 ounces broccoli
- 1 onion or leek, diced
- 1–2 tablespoons olive oil
- 1 red bell pepper, diced
- 8 ounces mushrooms, sliced
- pinch salt and pepper
- 12 large eggs
- 1 cup ricotta (or sour cream)
- 1 cup heavy cream (or sour cream)
- 1/2 teaspoon salt
- 1/2 teaspoon pepper
- 1/2 cup fresh basil (save some for garnish)
- 1–2 cups chopped baby spinach
- 1–2 cups grated mozzarella (or other melty cheese-cheddar, jack, or crumbled goat cheese)

Instructions

1. Preheat oven to 350F

2. Make the veggie filling: Cut the broccoli into small florets and steam until just tender, let cool. At the same time, saute the onion or leek in olive oil, 3-4 minutes, over medium heat. Add the peppers and mushrooms and season with salt and pepper. Keep sauteing until tender.

3. Make the custard: While the veggies are cooking whisk (or blend in a blender) the eggs with the ricotta, cream, salt and pepper. (Most any combo of ricotta, sour cream and cream will work here- 2 cups total.)

4. Assemble the frittata: Grease a deep 9 x 13-inch baking dish or 12-inch skillet. Pour 1/2 of the egg mixture in the bottom. Add the cooked veggies (you should have roughly 6 cups). Add the basil, spinach and cheese and pour in the remaining egg mixture. Give the veggies and little swirl so egg mixture is incorporated.

5. Bake: in the middle of the oven until the center is puffed and the frittata is nice and golden about 1 hour. Check at 30-40 minutes and tent with foil if getting too dark.

6. You'll know frittata is done with it puffs slightly at the very center and is not too wobbly.

7. Let stand 5 minutes before serving.

8. Leftovers keep 4 days in the fridge.

Prep Time: 20 Minutes

Cook Time: 65 Minutes

Servings: 8

Ingredients

- 1 loaf crusty sourdough or french bread, about 8 cups cubed
- 4–5 slices bacon (optional)
- 1 tablespoon oil
- 1 onion – very thinly sliced into rings
- 1–2 Tablespoons butter
- 1 pound of mushrooms sliced
- 3 Tablespoons fresh thyme leaves
- 10 large eggs
- 1 1/2 cups whole milk (or half and half)
- 1 cup sour cream
- 1 teaspoon salt
- 1/2 teaspoon pepper
- 4–6 ounces goat cheese
- thyme sprigs for garnish.
- 1 1/2 cups grated gruyere, jack, mozzerella cheese

Instructions

1. Preheat oven to 400F

2. Cut bread in to ¾ inch cubes and lay on a baking sheet and toast in the oven 10 minutes.

3. If adding bacon, spread out on a foil lined baking sheet and bake in the oven 20 minutes or until crisp. (Blot, then cut into small pieces)

4. In a large skillet, heat oil over medium high heat. Add thinly sliced onions. Saute, mixing often for 2-3 minutes, then turn heat down to medium low, continuing to cook until golden and tender, about 10 minutes. In another large skillet, heat butter over medium heat. Add sliced mushrooms and cook until tender, about 10 minutes. Add fresh thyme and a generous 3 finger pinch of salt and pepper, and cook off any liquid. Add the caramelized onions to the mushrooms and set aside.

5. In a medium bowl, whisk eggs, milk, sour cream, salt and pepper.

6. In a large bowl, add the toasted cubed bread. To this add the mushroom-onion-thyme mixture and bacon crumbles if using. Add the grated cheese and ⅔ of the crumbled goat cheese (saving the rest for the top) and gently mix.

7. Pour in the eggs and give a gentle stir. Let stand 5 minutes.

8. Stir again and pour into a well greased 4 quart baking dish. (At this point you could refrigerate overnight).

9. Cover with foil and place the 400 F oven and bake 35 minutes, Uncover, lower heat to 375 F and continue baking 20-30 more minutes until puffed and golden. During the last 10 minutes of baking, scatter the remaining goat cheese over the top and let it melt.

10. Garnish with a few thyme sprigs.

Prep Time: 10 Minutes

Cook Time: 25 Minutes

Servings: 12

Ingredients

- 6 large eggs
- 1 1/4 cup cottage cheese (full fat 4%)
- 1 1/4 cup shredded cheese- gruyere, cheddar, mozzarella, pepper jack, etc
- 1/4 teaspoon salt
- 1/4 teaspoon pepper
- 1 roasted bell pepper, sliced or diced (from a jar, or sub-canned green chilies, drained)
- 1/4– 1/2 cup fresh basil, ribbons (or sub cilantro or dill)
- optional: 6-12 cherry tomatoes, cut in half
- optional: 3 tablespoons parmesan

Instructions

1. Preheat oven to 300F. Place a pan of water 1/4 inch deep, on the lower rack to create steam. (see notes)
2. Grease a standard, non-stick muffin tin with olive oil. If not using non-stick, use muffin liners.
3. Place the eggs, cottage cheese, shredded cheese, salt and pepper in a blender and blend until silky smooth.
4. Pour and divide the batter into the greased muffin tins-to about 3/4 full.
5. Add the roasted pepper and basil to the top, stirring some down a bit. Top with a cherry tomato and sprinkle lightly with parmesan cheese.
6. Place the egg bites on the middle rack (over the pan with water) and bake until the egg bites are set and golden, about 20-24 minutes. Be doubly sure the center ones are set– they usually take 1-2 minutes longer than the ones on the edges.
7. Let cool 5- 10 minutes, loosen the edges with a knife, and carefully scoop them out with a spoon.
8. These will keep up to 4 days in the fridge or can be frozen and reheated.

Prep Time: 20 Minutes

Cook Time: 30 Minutes

Servings: 12

Ingredients

- 3 cups pastry flour (or sub-AP flour), spooned and leveled
- 1/2 teaspoon baking soda
- 2 1/2 teaspoons baking powder
- 1 teaspoon salt
- 3/4 cup cold butter (12 tablespoons, 1 1/2 sticks, or 6 ounces)
- 1 cup toasted pecans
- 1/2 cup cream (or half and half), more as needed
- 1/2 cup sour cream (or creme fraise, buttermilk or full-fat yogurt)
- 1/4 cup maple syrup
- 2 teaspoons vanilla

Maple glaze:

- 3 tablespoons maple syrup

- 1/2 cup powdered sugar

- 1/8 teaspoon salt

Instructions

1. Preheat oven 350 F oven

2. In a large bowl whisk together flour, baking soda, baking powder, and salt. Cut cold butter into thin slices and add to flour. (You could also freeze and grate). Using a pastry cutter, or two knives, begin cutting butter into smaller pieces into the flour. Feel free to use your fingers, breaking apart the butter into pieces no bigger than a pea. Having ununiform pieces is nice here. Add the pecans.

3. Whisk cream, sour cream, maple and vanilla in a small bowl. Stir this into the flour mixutre. Give it a few extra stirs, and if needed, add a few splashes of cream (a tablespoon at a time) until the mixture forms a shaggy ball and all the loose flour is incorporated.

4. Place on a floured surface. Give the dough just a few kneads (15 seconds) then form a ball.

5. Flatten into a 7-8 inch disk or 6×9 inch rectangle, and shore up the edges, using a dough scraper or chef's

knife- so edges are straight up and down, and the disk is the same thickness throughout. Feel free to tuck more pecans into the top (just for looks).

6. Cut into 8-12 equal pieces. Place on a parchment-lined sheet pan, 2-3 inches apart.

7. Bake until beautifully golden, puffed and internal temp reaches 200F (I highly recommend checking). Larger scones may take 30-35 minutes, smaller scones may take 20 minutes. So watch like a hawk!

8. While the scones are baking, make the Maple Glaze: in a little pot, heat the maple syrup. When warm, whisk in the powdered sugar until smooth. Add a pinch of salt. Turn off heat, leave on stove.

9. When the scones are done, let them cool for 15-20 minutes, then reheat the glaze and spoon a little over each one.

Prep Time: 15 Minutes

Cook Time: 20 Minutes

Servings: 8

Ingredients

- 1 loaf country sourdough bread, sliced into 3/4″ slices (or challah, brioche -softer airy bread will get the fluffiest-depends on the texture you prefer)
- 4 eggs
- 1 cup half and half
- 3 tablespoons maple syrup
- 1 teaspoon orange zest, about 1 medium orange worth
- 1 1/2 teaspoons cinnamon
- 1/2 teaspoon cardamom
- 1/4 teaspoon allspice
- 1/2 teaspoon nutmeg
- 1/4 teaspoon salt
- 4 tablespoons butter
- Berry Compote
- 3 cups berries, fresh preferred but frozen works too
- 1/4 cup maple syrup

- 3 tablespoons orange juice
- 1 tablespoon cornstarch
- tiny pinch of salt

Instructions

1. Whisk together the eggs, half and half, maple syrup, orange zest, cinnamon, cardamom, allspice, nutmeg and salt until completely smooth. Use an immersion blender if needed. Pour into a shallow container. (A rectangular pyrex works great to do several at the same time.)

2. Dip the slices of bread into the custard, letting it soak for 2-5 minutes on each side. (This will depend on the type of bread you use and how quickly it soaks up the custard.) Transfer to a rack placed over a pan and let excess drip off.

3. Heat a skillet to medium low. When the pan is fully heated, add 1/2 tablespoon of butter, as it melts place a soaked slice into the pan. Cooking for about 3 minutes per side, letting it get golden and slightly puffy in the center. Add more butter as needed.

4. Berry Compote

5. Bring maple syrup and 1 cup of the berries to a low bowl in a sauce pan. Let simmer for 2 minutes, mashing the berries a little with the back of a spoon to break down a bit.

6. Mix orange juice with cornstarch and a pinch of salt until perfectly smooth. Whisk into the maple berry mixture stirring all the while. Continue stirring until thick and bubbly, 2-3 minutes. Remove from heat.

7. Stir in the remaining 2 cups of berries.

8. To Serve: Top the French Toast with berry compote and yogurt cream. (More butter and maple syrup is optional of course!)

Prep Time: 15 Minutes

Cook Time: 10 Minutes

Servings: 1

Ingredients

- 1/2 cup regular rolled oats
- 1/3 cup coconut milk or yogurt (or use vegan yogurt)
- 1/4 cup water or milk (your favorite: almond milk, hemp milk, etc.)
- 1/4 teaspoon vanilla extract
- 2 teaspoons maple syrup
- pinch of sea salt
- 2 teaspoons chia seeds (optional)
- 4 servings
- 2 cups regular rolled oats
- 1 1/3 cups coconut milk or yogurt
- 1 cup water or milk (your favorite: almond milk, hemp milk, etc.)
- 1 t vanilla extract
- 2–3 tablespoons maple syrup
- 1/2 teaspoon sea salt

- 2 1/2 tablespoons chia seeds

Additions:

- Add overnight: raisins, currants, dates, orange or lemon zest, chocolate chips, nut butter
- Add morning of: fresh fruit, spices, toasted nuts and seeds, cocoa nibs, toasted unsweetened coconut, a dollop of Greek yogurt.
- Favorite combinations:
- almond or peanut butter, banana, cocoa nibs, a sprinkle of cinnamon
- yogurt, blueberry, lemon zest, cardamom, almond
- dates and superfood crunch mix
- raisins, apple, cinnamon
- orange zest, peach, pecan, cinnamon
- dried cherries and almond butter
- tahini, cocoa powder, coconut flakes and dates

Instructions

1. Mix all ingredients together.
2. Place in a sealed container.
3. Store in the fridge overnight.

4. Top with desired toppings, add yogurt and more milk
    if needed.

Prep Time: 15 Minutes

Cook Time: 10 Minutes

Servings: 4

Ingredients

Chia Yogurt Base Mix:

- 1/3 cup chia seeds
- 1/2 cup boiled hot water
- 3 tablespoons honey (maple, coconut sugar)
- 2 teaspoon vanilla
- pinch of sea salt
- 1 1/2 cups greek yogurt (or vegan yogurt)
- 1 1/2 cups nut milk (almond, hemp, oat, soy, etc.)

3 optional flavors:

- Golden Glow
- 1 cup chia yogurt base mix
- 1/2 teaspoon turmeric
- 1/2 teaspoon ginger
- 1/8 teaspoon orange zest
- fresh cubed mango

- 2 dates
- toasted coconut flakes
- Mexican Cacao Dream
- 1 cup chia yogurt base mix
- 2 teaspoons raw chocolate powder
- 1/4 teaspoon cinnamon
- 1/8 teaspoon ancho chili powder
- 2 teaspoon maple syrup
- 2 teaspoon cacao nibs
- banana slices
- Berry Happy
- 1 cup chia yogurt base mix
- 1/4 teaspoon ground cardamom
- fresh raspberries
- fresh blueberries
- fresh strawberries
- sliced almonds

Instructions

1. In a quart jar, mix chia seeds and hot water. Let sit about 5 minutes. This starts hydrating the chia seed more quickly.

2. Stir in vanilla, honey (or maple) and pinch of salt.

3. Add greek yogurt and nut milk. Whisk to thoroughly combine. (At this point you could divide into 4 smaller jars.)

4. At this stage it will keep in the refrigerator for 4-5 days.

5. Add preferred flavor and fruits to serve. Refrigerate at least an hour before serving.

11. Middle Eastern Eggplant Wrap

Prep Time: 10 Minutes

Cook Time: 30 Minutes

Servings: 2- 4

Ingredients

- 1 small eggplant (1 pound)
- olive oil, salt and pepper
- Kale Slaw (or make the Everyday Kale Slaw and add fresh herbs)
- 6–7 lacinato (or tuscan) kale leaves – 2 cups shredded (packed)
- 1 bunch italian parsley
- handful mint leaves
- ¼ cup finely diced onion
- 2 tablespoons olive oil
- 2 tablespoons lemon juice
- ¼ teaspoon salt
- optional additions- sliced tomato, radishes, cucumber, feta, yogurt

- Quick tahini sauce (or sub store bought, tahini sauce or baba ganoush)
- 2 tablespoons tahini paste
- 3 tablespoons hot tap water
- 1 tablespoon lemon juice
- ⅛ tablespoon salt
- 1 minced garlic clove
- 2– 4 wraps or tortillas (feel free to use gluten free) 8-10 inch

Instructions

1. Preheat oven to 425F
2. Slice eggplant into ¼ inch thick disks.
3. Brush each side with olive oil and season with salt and pepper. Place on a parchment lined sheet pan and roast the oven for 25-30 minutes, flipping over after 20 minutes. While they are baking, make the slaw filling and sauce.
4. Thinly slice the kale into thin ribbons, stacking them first then slicing(see photo). Place in a bowl. Finally chop the parsley and mint, thin stems are ok. Add to the bowl along with the onion. Toss with olive oil, lemon juice, salt and pepper. You want this to be quite

"juicy", so if needed add a little more oil and lemon juice in equal portions. You can add radishes and/ or tomatoes here if you want or sprinkle them over top of the wrap.

5. Whisk together the tahini sauce ingredients in a small bowl.

6. Lightly warm or toast the tortilla or wrap. Spread the inside with tahini sauce. Top with warm eggplant and a huge mound of the dressed greens. Top with tomatoes, radishes and feta if you like.

7. This recipe make 2 enormous wraps or 4 smaller ones. Or three medium ones. ⍰

8. Notes: For even more flavor, grill the eggplant during the warm months. Both the eggplant and the kale slaw can be made ahead and refrigerated.

Prep Time: 15 Minutes

Cook Time: 08 Minutes

Servings: 4

Ingredients

- 1/2 cup shredded coconut, toasted
- 1/3 cup cashews, toasted
- 1 14 ounce can chickpeas, drained (1 1/2 cups cooked chickpeas)
- 8–10 dates, chopped small
- 1 cup celery, diced
- 1/2 cup apple, chopped
- ¼ cup red onion, finely diced (or sub green onion)
- ¼ cup cilantro, chopped (or sub scallions)
- 1 tablespoon orange zest (optional)
- 3–4 tablespoons Vegenaise, mayo or vegan mayo
- 1 tablespoon maple (or honey, agave, or alternative sweetener)
- 2 teaspoons apple cider vinegar
- 2–3 teaspoons yellow curry powder (start with two, add more to taste, some brands are spicy)

- 1/4 teaspoon salt, more to taste
- 1/4 teaspoon pepper

Instructions

1. Toast cashews and coconut over low heat, until golden and fragrant.
2. Place chickpeas in a medium bowl and add celery, apple, dates, onion, cilantro and zest.
3. Mix in the vegan mayo, maple and vinegar, until well combined. Add the curry powder, salt and pepper. Toss in the toasted coconut and cashews. Mix.
4. Taste, and add more salt if needed. Feel free to add more curry powder or a pinch of cayenne for more heat or flavor.
5. Serving options:
6. Wrap up in a whole wheat tortilla (or pita) with a handful of spinach, greens or sprouts
7. Serve over a bed of greens lightly dressed with olive oil, salt and lemon or AC vinegar
8. Serve in a halved, salted, avocado.
9. Serve in lettuce cups

Prep Time: 15 Minutes

Cook Time: 30 Minutes

Servings: 6

Ingredients

Preserved Lemon Dressing:

- 1/4 cup preserved lemons, finely chopped
- 1/4 cup olive oil
- 1/4 cup lemon juice
- 2 garlic cloves, finely minced
- 1/2 teaspoon salt
- 1/2 teaspoon pepper
- 1/2 teaspoon sumac (optional)

Chickpea Quinoa Salad:

- 3/4 cup quinoa (dry, uncooked)
- 1 1/2 cups water
- 1 15-ounce can chickpeas, rinsed and drained (1 1/2 cups cooked chickpeas)
- 1/2 cup red onion, finely chopped (see notes)
- 1 English cucumber, diced (2 cups)

- 1 bell pepper (yellow is nice) diced
- 1 cup cherry or grape tomatoes, halved (or chopped radish)
- 1/4 cup kalamata olives, chopped or halved
- 1/2 cup flat-leaf parsley, chopped
- 1/4 cup dill, chopped (or sub mint, or use both!)
- Other optional additions: avocado, feta, radishes

Instructions

1. Place quinoa, water and pinch of salt in a medium pot, bring to a boil, cover, simmer on low 12-15 minutes until all the water is gone. Uncover, fluff, cool slightly.
2. Make the dressing, by mixing all in a bowl.
3. Prep all the veggies. If sensitive to onions, dice, then soak in cold salted water while you chop the rest.
4. Place the chickpeas, onions, cucumber, bell pepper, tomatoes, olives, dill and parsley to a large bowl. Add the quinoa and dressing and give a good toss.
5. Taste, adjust salt and lemon to your liking. If making ahead, taste once more right before serving as the quinoa and chickpeas have a tendency to soak up the salt and lemon, so you might want to add a little more.

Prep Time: 15 Minutes

Cook Time: 30 Minutes

Servings: 8

Ingredients

- 2 tablespoons olive oil
- one onion, diced
- 5–6 garlic cloves, rough chopped
- 3 carrots, diced (2 cups) (or sub other root veggies- yam or sweet potato, parsnips, celery root, sunchokes)
- 1 red bell pepper, diced
- 1 poblano pepper, diced (optional, for a subtle heat)
- one 14-ounce can diced tomatoes (or sub 1 1/2 cups diced tomatoes with juices)
- 4 cups veggie broth (or chicken broth)
- 1/2 teaspoon salt
- teaspoons cumin
- 1 teaspoon chili powder
- 1 teaspoon coriander
- 1 teaspoon cinnamon
- 1 teaspoon dried thyme (or add a few bay leaves)

- 1/2 teaspoon turmeric

- 1 teaspoon maple syrup (or honey)

- 3/4 cup red lentils (split lentils)

- 1/4 cup quinoa

optional addtions: 1/4 cup raisins

Garnish:

- fresh cilantro,parsley, scallions or mint, a squeeze of lemon or lime, a drizzle of olive oil (or swirl of yogurt) or even sliced avocado.

Instructions

1. Set Instant Pot (Pressure cooker) to saute function and heat the oil. Add the onion and garlic and saute 3-4 minutes, stirring until fragrant. Add the carrots, bell pepper and optional poblano and stir 2 minutes.

2. Add the diced tomatoes (and juices) and broth. Stir in the salt, cumin, chili powder, coriander, cinnamon, turmeric, thyme, and maple syrup. Stir in the split red lentils and the quinoa. You will be tempted to add more but don't. ▢ Give a good stir. At this point, you could also toss in 1/4 cup raisins (or add after).

3 Set instant pot to high pressure for 5 minutes. Manually release (cover the spout with a kitchen towel).

4 Taste, adjust salt if needed. For a bit of acid, a squeeze of lemon or lime is nice. The stew will thicken as it sits.

5 Serve this up with fresh radishes and herbs. Add a drizzle of olive oil (or for extra richness and a swirl of yogurt).

Prep Time: 15 Minutes

Cook Time: 10 Minutes

Servings: 4-6

Ingredients

- oz pasta like fusilli, torchetti, bow ties- something that hangs on to the bits and pieces
- 3 garlic cloves minced
- 1/4– 1/2 teaspoon red pepper flakes
- 2 tablespoons olive oil, divided
- 3/4 cup olive tapenade
- 2 cans good quality tuna, 5 oz (in olive oil preferred)
- 2 teaspoon lemon zest
- 2 cups fresh arugula
- 1/4 cup lemon juice
- 1 1/2 cups fresh tomatoes, chopped
- 1/2 cup fresh basil or parsley
- salt and pepper

Instructions

1. Cook pasta according to package directions in salted water. Do not rinse.

2. Make the Olive Tapenade.

3. Sauté garlic, pepper flakes, and olive oil for a few minutes until it smells fragrant and barely begins to color. Add olive tapenade, tuna and the oil, and lemon zest and heat to warm, about a minute.

4. Add hot pasta, arugula, lemon juice (start with 1/8 cup and add more to taste), stir to combine. Add tomatoes, sprinkle on fresh basil and add salt and pepper to taste.

Prep Time: 15 Minutes

Cook Time: 10 Minutes

Servings: 3

Ingredients

Pancakes:

- 1/2 cup water
- 1/2 cup rice flour
- 2 eggs
- 2 teaspoons gochujang hot pepper paste (see notes)
- 2 teaspoons mirin
- 1/4 teaspoon white pepper
- 1 teaspoon sea salt
- 1 medium zucchini, cut in thin strips or grated or spiralized
- 1 bunch scallions, slice in quarters long ways, creating strips about 4–5 inches long
- 1 tablespoon raw sesame seeds, untoasted
- avocado oil or other high heat cooking oil

Dipping Sauce:

- 2 tablespoons soy sauce

- 1 tablespoon rice vinegar

- 1 teaspoon sesame oil

- 1 teaspoon sugar, maple syrup or honey (optional)

- a pinch of red pepper flakes, if desired

Instructions

1   Mix together water, rice flour, eggs, gochujang, mirin, white pepper, and salt. Set aside to hydrate while you prepare the veggies.

2   Mix prepared veggies into the rice flour batter.

3   Heat a cast iron or other non-stick pan to medium high heat, oil the pan with a teaspoon or so of oil. Use tongs to place battered veggies onto the pan, spreading out so they are not piled on each other. Spoon on batter to fill in any holes. Keeping it thin and no bigger then 7 inches.

4   Sprinkle on a teaspoon of sesame seeds. Cook for 3 minutes per side. After flipping, press pancake down with a metal spatula to flatten and cook more evenly on the underside.

5   Serve with kimchi and dipping sauce.

Prep Time: 25 Minutes

Cook Time: 10 Minutes

Servings: 4

Ingredients

Quesadilla Filling:

- 2 tablespoons olive oil
- 1/2 an onion, diced (1 cup)
- 4 garlic cloves, rough chopped
- 4 cups finely chopped veggies: bell pepper, zucchini, summer squash, mushrooms, broccoli, sweet potato, corn, etc. (Chop the veggies small, so they cook faster!)
- 1/2 teaspoon salt
- 1 teaspoon dried oregano
- 1 teaspoon cumin
- 1 teaspoon coriander
- 1 teaspoon chili powder
- 1–2 cups chopped greens- beet greens, turnip greens, spinach, chard, etc.

- 1 cup black beans (cooked or canned)
- 2 tablespoons water
- 1/4 cup cilantro, chopped- optional
- 1 teaspoon lime zest- optional
- 4 x 10-12 inch tortillas (I used sundried tomato tortillas)
- ounces shredded cheese- Oaxacan string cheese, mozzarella, pepper jack, etc. (or sub vegan cheese)

Spicy Sour Cream:

- 1/4 cup sour cream (or yogurt)
- 2–3 tablespoons hot sauce (fermented hot sauce is great here)

Serve with:

- Pico De Gallo!

Instructions

1 Preheat the oven to 400F (or preheat grill to medium)

Make the Veggie Filling:

1   Heat oil in an extra-large skillet over medium-high heat. Add the onion and garlic, saute 3-4 minutes until fragrant. Lower heat to medium, and add the chopped veggies and salt. Stir occasionally until the veggies soften (check) and release their liquid, about 10 minutes (lower heat if need be). Add the oregano, cumin, coriander, chili powder and give a good stir. Add the chopped greens and black beans and a couple of tablespoons of water, and stir until the greens wilt 1-2 minutes. Turn heat off. Stir in optional cilantro and lime zest.

Assemble the Quesadillas:

1   Scatter 1/2 cup cheese over the whole tortilla. Add one cup of veggie filling over half of the tortilla. Fold the Tortilla in half so the filling is encased with cheese (see photo). Brush the outer side of the tortilla with oil, and place in a hot oven for 15 minutes. You can place the greased quesadilla directly on the oven grates, or on a parchment-lined sheet pan, flipping halfway through. Bake until tortilla is crispy and cheese is melty.

2   Cut each into 4 pieces and serve with the Spicy Sour Cream and Pico De Gallo

3   To make the spicy sour cream– simply mix a few
    tablespoons of hot sauce with the sour cream in a little
    bowl.

Prep Time: 25 Minutes

Cook Time: 2hrs 10 Minutes

Servings: 4

Ingredients

- large peaches (3–4 inches wide) save 1/4 cup for garnish
- large tomatoes (same size as peaches) save 1/4 cup for garnish
- 1/3 of an English cucumber, about 1 1/2 cups– save 1/4 cup for garnish
- 1/4 cup red onion, sliced, plus 1/4 cup for garnish
- 10 basil leaves, plus more for garnish
- 1 tablespoon olive oil
- 1/2 –1 teaspoon salt
- 1–2 teaspoons red wine vinegar, sherry vinegar, or champagne vinegar (or Apple Cider vinegar)
- cracked pepper to taste

Garnish:

- Finely diced peaches, tomato, cucumber and red onion, torn basil leaves, and pick one of the following: drizzle of olive oil, sliced avocado, burrata cheese (or ricotta or vegan ricotta).

- Feel free to add croutons or serve with crusty bread.

- I've also topped this with fresh crab.

Instructions

1 Quarter the peaches and tomatoes and set aside one wedge of each for your garnish.

2 Place the remaining peaches and tomatoes in a blender. Add the onion, cucumber, (setting aside garnish portions) basil, olive oil, 1/2 teaspoon salt, pepper and 1 teaspoon vinegar.

3 Blend until relatively smooth. Taste. Adjust salt and vinegar to your liking, find your perfect balance. If too peachy add more tomato! It should be tomato forward with hints of peach.

4 Chill at least 2 hours.

5 While chilling, chop up the garnish ingredients as finely as possible. Chill as well.

6 To serve, ladle the cold gazpacho into a bowl, sprinkle with garnishes- a crescent shape is pretty, or create

your own style. Drizzle with olive oil and add a dollop of burrata or ricotta. Scatter with torn basil leaves. Feel free to add croutons or serve with crusty bread.

Prep Time: 25 Minutes

Cook Time: 20 Minutes

Servings: 2

Ingredients

Cajun Vegan Ranch Dressing

- ⅓ cup vegan ranch dressing (or sub your favorite store-bought ranch)
- ½ –1 teaspoon cajun spice blend (or sub ¼ teaspoon paprika, and 1/4 teaspoon cayenne)
- Blackened Tempeh:
- 1 block tempeh
- 2–3 tablespoons Cajun Spice like Black Magic
- tablespoons olive oil

Salad

- 4–5 leaves of lacinato kale, tough stems removed (or use 3 cups pre-shredded kale)
- 1 teaspoon oil, pinch salt, lemon zest from ½ a lemon
- radishes, sliced (or sub cucumber slices... or ribbons are nice)

- 1 scallion, sliced

- 1 avocado, sliced

- ¼ cup pickled onions (optional)

- cilantro leaves (optional)

Optional add-ons:

- Sprouts or microgreens, cooked quinoa, large whole wheat tortillas, sauerkraut.

Instructions

Make the dressing:

1 Stir the cajun spice into the dressing, starting conservatively. Taste, and add more to taste. You want it bold!

Prepare the tempeh:

1 Add the tempeh, whole to a sauté pan of generously salted water, just enough to cover it. Let simmer gently 8-10 minutes to help soften and reduce bitterness. Slice it into ½ inch wide slices and generously coat each side with Cajun Spices.Pan-sear the tempeh in a little oil, until crispy and heated through. Set aside.

Make the salad:

1   Stack the kale (removing any thick stems) and cut into thin ribbons. Place in a bowl and add a teaspoon or two of olive oil (just enough to barely coat) a generous pinch salt and the lemon zest. Massage with your fingers until tender.

2   To the kale add the radishes, scallion, pickled onion and avocado. Toss with some of the Vegan Ranch dressing, enough to coat. (You can also keep everything separate, especially if making grain bowls)

3   Either divide the salad among bowls or place in warm, whole wheat tortillas, topped with the blackened tempeh and sprouts.

4   The salad is hearty enough that it will taste good the next day.

Prep Time: 15 Minutes

Cook Time: 25 Minutes

Servings: 6-8

Ingredients

- tablespoons olive oil
- 1 large onion, diced small
- 1 1/2 cups carrots, diced small
- 1 1/2 cups celery, diced
- 1 red or green bell pepper, diced
- 1 cup diced sweet potato or parsnips (or leave out)
- 4–6 fat cloves of garlic, rough chopped
- tablespoons mild chili powder
- 1 tablespoon dried oregano
- 1 teaspoons cumin
- 1 teaspoon coriander
- 1 teaspoon smoked paprika
- 1 teaspoon kosher salt, divided
- 1/4 teaspoon cayenne, or ground chipotle
- ⅛ teaspoon cinnamon (optional)

- 14-ounce can of diced tomatoes, with juices, or 1 1/2 cups fresh tomatoes, diced (with juices)
- x 14-ounce cans beans – any assortment of black, pinto, kidney or etc. (drain and rinse) about 4.5 cups cooked beans.
- 1 cup of veggie broth
- 1 tablespoon soy sauce (or GF Liquid Amino's) or sub 1-2 veggie bullion paste or cubes
- tablespoons tomato paste
- Teaspoons dark cocoa powder, or one square of dark chocolate (optional, but good!)
- 1–2 teaspoons maple syrup (or brown sugar) more to taste

Optional:

- add crumbled or ground plant-based meat, like soy crumbles.

Optional:

- 1/2 cup ground walnuts or ground pecans

Optional Garnishes

- avocado, pickled jalapeno, pickled onions, chopped tomatoes, radishes, cilantro, scallions, vegan sour cream, vegan cheddar or a drizzle of olive oil

Instructions

1 Dice the onion, and saute in a large dutch oven over medium-high heat with a few tablespoons of olive oil, until fragrant and golden. Lower heat to medium, add the carrots, celery and garlic, and saute 5 more minutes.

2 Chop the bell pepper and sweet potato and add to the pot, season with ½ teaspoon salt and continue cooking for 10 minutes, or until veggies are just tender, stirring occasionally.

3 While this happening, line up your spices, rinse and drain the beans. If using fresh tomatoes, dice them saving the juices.

4 When the veggies are just tender add the spices – chili powder, cumin, coriander, oregano, smoked paprika, cayenne, cinnamon. Toast the spices in the pot for 1-2 minutes to bring their flavors forward. Add the tomatoes (with their juices), beans and veggie broth.

5 Add the remaining 1/2 teaspoon salt, stir, and then cover with a lid, and simmer gently on medium low heat, for 10 more minutes or until veggies are fork-tender.

6 Stir in the tomato paste, soy sauce , chocolate and maple syrup. Add the optional ground walnuts. The

ground nuts add depth and also thicken the chili. If leaving them out, you could blend 1-2 cups of chili in the blender and return this to the pot to thicken.

7   Taste, adjust, adding more salt, spices, or maple syrup as needed.

8   Serve with any of the following: fresh cilantro, diced avocado, scallions, pickled jalapeno, hot sauce, sliced radishes, pickled onions, vegan sour cream or vegan grated cheddar, or a drizzle of olive oil.

21. Brazilian Fish Stew – Moqueca

Prep Time: 20 Minutes

Cook Time: 35 Minutes

Servings: 4

Ingredients

Fish:

- 1 – 1 1/2 pounds firm white fish- Halibut, Black Cod, Sea Bass (thicker cuts are best)
- ½ teaspoon salt
- one lime- zest and juice

Stew/ Sauce:

- 2–3 tablespoons coconut or olive oil (or use Dende – Brazillian Red Palm oil for the best flavor!)
- 1 onion- finely diced (red, white or yellow)
- 1/2 teaspoon salt
- 1 cup carrot, diced
- 1 red bell pepper, diced
- garlic cloves- rough chopped

- 1/2 jalapeno, finely diced
- 1 tablespoon tomato paste
- teaspoons paprika
- 1 teaspoon ground cumin (or whole seed)
- 1 cup fish or chicken stock
- 1 1/2 cups tomatoes, diced (preferably fresh)
- 14 ounce can coconut milk (liquid and solids)
- more salt to taste
- ½ cup chopped cilantro, scallions or Italian parsley
- squeeze of lime
- Serve over cilantro rice, basmati rice, black rice or everyday quinoa.

Instructions

1 Rinse and pat dry the fish and cut into 2 inch peices. Place in a bowl. Add salt, zest from half the lime and 1 tablespoon lime juice. Massage lightly to coat all pieces well. Set aside.

2 In a large saute pan, heat the olive oil over medium high heat. Add onion and salt, and sauté 2-3 minutes. Turn heat down to medium, add carrot, bell pepper, garlic and jalapeno and cook 4-5 more minutes. Add tomato paste, spices and stock. Mix and bring to a

simmer and add tomatoes. Cover and simmer gently on medium low for 5 mintues or until carrots are tender.

3   Add the coconut milk and taste and add more salt if necessary.

4   Nestle the fish in the stew and simmer gently until it's cooked through, about 4-6 minutes. Spoon the flavorful coconut broth over the fish and cook until desired doneness or longer for thicker pieces. (You can also finish this in a 350F oven).

5   Taste and adjust salt and squeeze with lime.

6   To serve, serve over rice, sprinkle with cilantro or scallions and a squeeze of lime.

7   Drizzle with a little olive oil if you like.

Prep Time: 20 Minutes

Cook Time: 15 Minutes

Servings: 2

Ingredients

- 1 block tofu- organic, extra firm, drained
- tablespoons olive oil or coconut oil
- 1/4 teaspoon salt
- 1/4 teaspoon pepper
- 1/4 cup BBQ Sauce (aim for one without high fructose corn syrup, or make your own)
- 1 teaspoon chili paste or sriracha
- soft buns, (like brioche buns) toasted
- Avocado- optional, messy but good. ⍰

Creamy Cilantro Slaw:

- ounces shredded cabbage- about 3 cups packed
- 1/4 cup cilantro, chopped
- 1/4 cup red onion, thinly sliced
- 3–4 tablespoons vegan mayo (or regular mayo) or make your own

- 1 tablespoon vinegar- Apple Cider or white, more to taste

- 1/4 teaspoon salt

Instructions

1 Drain the block of tofu, pat dry, and cut into one-inch-thick slabs. Trim if needed to fit the bun. You can get 2, maybe 3 out of one block. Pat dry again.

2 Heat a skillet over medium-high heat. Add oil, and sprinkle the salt and pepper over the oil. Once the pepper is fragrant, carefully add the tofu. Sear until crispy and deeply golden- do not move it around in the pan, let it develop a crust, so it will release itself. Lower heat if splattering- this will take about 12 minutes.

3 Mix the BBQ sauce and red chili paste in a small bowl and set aside.

4 Place the shredded cabbage in a medium bowl, add onions and cilantro, mayo, vinegar, and salt, and toss to combine well. Taste. It should be creamy, tangy and flavorful. Feel free to add more vinegar, salt or mayo to attain this. All mayos are different!

5 Toast the buns and slice the avocado.

6   Once the tofu is nice and crispy, lower the heat to low, and add the bbq sauce mixture, coating the tofu well. I use all the sauce. Let it caramelize just slightly in the pan, and turn the heat off.

7   Assemble the Sandwich. Spread more mayo on the bottom bun if you like, add the hot tofu, and top with cool slaw and a few slices of avocado.

8   EAT immediately.

Prep Time: 15 Minutes

Cook Time: 30 Minutes

Servings: 5

Ingredients

- tablespoons olive oil (or butter)
- cups sliced leeks (one extra large leek)
- garlic cloves, rough chopped
- sage leaves, chopped
- 1 cup Arborio rice or short-grain Spanish rice
- heaping cups butternut squash, cubed
- 1/4 cup white wine (or skip it)
- cups veggie stock or chicken stock or broth (or water and one teaspoon or cube veggie bouillon)
- 1/2 teaspoon salt
- 1/8 teaspoon white pepper (or sub black pepper to taste)
- 1/2 teaspoon nutmeg the nutmeg makes this- don't leave it out!
- 2–3 handfuls baby spinach or chopped kale

OPTIONAL:

- 1/4 – 1/2 cup parmesan, pecorino, manchego, goat cheese, vegan cheese or cashew cheese – or the leave cheese out and use LEEK OIL for garnish. Or stir in 1-2 tablespoons of butter or ghee, or a drizzle of olive oil.

Optional:

- Maple Glazed Pecans

Instructions

1. Slice and rinse leeks, separating rings (rinsing will help them to soften faster).
2. Set Instant Pot to the "Saute" function.
3. Heat oil in the instant pot, add the rinsed leeks and stir for 2 minutes. Add garlic, sage and rice, stir for 2 minutes.
4. Add butternut squash, and keep stirring for a couple of minutes, until there is a bit of browning on the bottom of the instant pot.
5. Add the wine and scrape up the browned bits- a wooden spoon is good for this. Let all the wine cook off, about 2-3 minutes. Add the stock or broth. Scrape

up more browned bits. Add the salt, pepper and nutmeg, and give a good stir.

6   Seal the instant pot and pressure cook on HIGH for 6 minutes. Naturally, release for 5 minutes, then manually release.

7   While the Instant pot is going you could make the leek oil and/or the maple glazed pecans.

8   Stir the risotto, adding the spinach and cheese or butter if you like, or leave them out. As the butternut breaks down a bit, it will add a nice natural creaminess to the risotto.

9   Garnish with optional leek oil or maple glazed pecans.

Prep Time: 15 Minutes

Cook Time: 35 Minutes

Servings: 4-7

Ingredients

- tablespoons olive oil
- 1 large onion, diced
- 1 1/2 cup carrots, small diced
- 1 1/2 cups celery diced
- 4–6 cloves garlic, rough chopped
- 1 1/2 teaspoon salt
- 1/2 teaspoon pepper
- 1/4 teaspoon chili flakes- optional
- 1 tablespoon fresh oregano or thyme (or 2 teaspoons dried Italian herbs)
- 1/3 cup tomato paste
- Generous splash red wine (optional) 1/4 cup-ish
- 1 1/4 cup black caviar lentils (or other small lentils- see notes)
- medium tomatoes, diced with juices (or sub a 14-ounce can of diced tomatoes or crushed tomatoes)

- 1/2 cups veggie stock or broth (or sub water plus 2-3 boullion cubes)
- 3/4 cup hemp seeds, or crushed toasted walnuts or pecans
- teaspoons balsamic vinegar

Instructions

1. Heat oil in a large pot or dutch oven over medium-high heat. Add the onion and saute for 2-3 minutes stirring until fragrant. Lower heat to medium, then add the carrots, celery, garlic, salt, pepper, chili flakes, and herbs. Saute 7-8 minutes, stirring.

2. Add the tomato paste, browning it just a bit in the pan (this will deepen the flavor), then deglaze with wine if you want, scraping up any brown bits. Once most of the wine has cooked off add the tomatoes and their juices, cook them down for just a few minutes.

3. Add the lentils, veggie stock and hemp seeds or walnuts. Bring to a boil, cover tightly, lower heat to low, and simmer gently 20-25 minutes, or until the lentils are tender. Uncover.

4. Continue cooking uncovered until most of the liquid has cooked off. Stir in the balsamic vinegar, taste, and

adjust salt, pepper, vinegar and chili flakes to your liking. Keep in mind, you want this just slightly salty if tossing with pasta.

5   Serve this tossed with your favorite pasta or serve it over this creamy polenta or this Instant Pot Polenta. Sprinkle with optional pecorino cheese... or try this Vegan Cheesy Sprinkle!

Prep Time: 25 Minutes

Cook Time: 45 Minutes

Servings: 3-4

Ingredients

- 8–10 ounces orecchiette pasta, cooked in salted water, according to package directions.

Carrot Miso Sauce:

- shallots, rough chopped (or 1/2 an onion)
- 4–6 garlic cloves, rough chopped
- tablespoons olive oil
- heaping cups carrots, thinly sliced (3 medium carrots)
- cups water
- 1/4 cup raw cashews (or sub raw hemp seeds)
- 1/4 teaspoon salt
- 1/4 teaspoon pepper
- tablespoons White Miso Paste
- Carrot Top Gremolata (optional, but tasty)
- 1/2 cup carrot tops (tender leaves) packed or sub 1/2 cup more Italian Parsley

- 1/2 cup Italian parsley

- 1 fat garlic clove

- 1 tablespoon lemon zest (zest from one med lemon)

- 1/4 teaspoon salt

- 1/3 cup– 1/2 cup olive oil (make sure it is not bitter-
  taste it!)

- 1–2 teaspoons lemon juice.

Instructions

Cook Pasta:

1   Set 6-8 cups salted water to boil for pasta, and cook
    according to directions.

Cook The Sauce:

1   Heat oil in a medium pot, over medium heat. Saute
    shallot and garlic until fragrant and golden, about 5
    minutes, stirring often. Add carrots, cashews, water,
    salt and pepper and bring to a boil. Cover, lower heat
    to low and simmer gently until carrots are fork-
    tender, about 15 minutes. Stir in the 3 tablespoons of
    miso (it doesn't need to dissolve fully) and let cool for
    5-10 minutes.

2   While the carrots simmer make the optional Carrot Top Gremolata and Toasted Panko or Bread Crumbs

BLEND THE CARROT MISO SAUCE:

1   Once the carrots are tender and slightly cooled, place all in a high-speed blender, covering tightly with a kitchen towel, blend on the lowest setting, gradually increasing speed, until fully blended, creamy and silky smooth about 1- 1 1/2 minutes. Take your time here and get it SMOOTH!!!

2   Drain the pasta and pour the sauce over the pasta, gently warming if needed. Taste and adjust salt. (If you didn't salt your pasta water, chances are you'll need salt.)

3   Divide among bowls, and sprinkle with toasted bread crumbs and spoon the flavorful Carrot Top Gremolata over top.

Prep Time: 45 Minutes

Cook Time: 1hrs 45 Minutes

Servings: 8

Ingredients

- 1/2 lbs potatoes (Yukon gold, red, or any thin-skinned) (OR use 5 cups leftover mashed potatoes, with curry powder)
- tablespoons, ghee, butter, vegan butter (ghee tastes the BEST)
- 1/2 cup plain yogurt (or sour cream)
- 1/2 cup milk(or nut milk), half and half or heavy cream
- 1 teaspoon salt, more to taste
- 1/2 teaspoon pepper
- 1–2 teaspoons yellow curry powder, more to taste

Filling:

- 1/2 cups cooked lentils (3/4 cup -1 cup dry)
- tablespoons ghee, or olive oil
- 1 large onion, diced

- cloves garlic, rough chopped
- cups diced carrot, (2–3 carrots)
- cups diced celery (2–3 ribs)
- teaspoons garam masala, more to taste
- 1 teaspoon cumin
- 1 teaspoon coriander
- 1 teaspoon salt
- 1/2 teaspoon pepper
- teaspoons dried fenugreek leaves
- 1 cup veggie broth
- 1 cup frozen peas (or corn, or green beans- or use fresh)

Gravy:

- tablespoon ghee or olive oil
- 1 teaspoon cumin seeds
- 1 teaspoon fennel seeds
- tablespoons flour (or gf flour)
- 1 1/4 cups warm veggie broth

optional garnish:

- scallions, chives, or cilantro

Instructions

1. Preheat oven to 350F

2. Cook Potatoes: Cut potatoes in one-inch slices (if small, just in half) and place in a large pot. Cover with one-inch salted water. Bring to a boil, lower heat, cover and simmer until very tender about 20-25 minutes.

3. Cook lentils: Set lentils to cook in salted water (unless cooked already – and you could absolutely do this ahead) about 20-25 minutes (see notes) simmer until tender, but not falling apart, al dente.

4. Make the filling: In a large 10-12 inch ovenproof skillet (or wide, shallow dutch oven) -heat the ghee over medium high heat and saute the onion 2-3 minutes, lower heat to med, add garlic, saute 2 mintues, add carrots, celery, cook 5-7 mintues. Add salt, cumin, coriander, fenugreek leaves and garam masala.

5. Add broth. Bring to a simmer, cover and simmer on med low, until carrots are cooked through about 7-8 minutes.

6. While this is simmering, MAKE THE GRAVY: Over medium heat, in a little pot, simmer the whole seeds (cumin seeds and fennel seeds) in ghee or oil until

fragrant and golden. Add flour, whisking, stirring and toasting the flour one minute. Gradually whisk in the warm veggie broth. Cook until slightly thickened. Add this gravy to the filling, along with the peas and drained lentils. Mix to combine.

7   Taste the filling and adjust salt and pepper. Add more garam masala if you like. The filling should have thick stew-like, saucy consistency. If too dry, add a splash of broth or water. If too watery, simmer off some of that liquid. If the filling is too watery, the mashed potatoes will sink.

8   Mash the potatoes: Drain the potatoes (saving some hot potato water) return to the same pot and mash with the 3-4 tablespoons ghee and yogurt. If potatoes seem dry or too stiff, add a little warm potato water to loosen. If you want extra richness a little milk, nut milk, half and half, or whipping cream is nice. I add about ½ cup. (Adding more yogurt will make these too tangy.) Season with salt, pepper and curry powder. Mash and whip until relatively smooth and light and fluffy. Taste and adjust salt.

9   ASSEMBLE: Place 8 big dollops over the lentils stew and fill in the spaces with smaller spoonfuls, carefully

spreading out, maybe making a pattern with the back of the spoon, like frosting a cake.

10 Place in the oven until golden and bubbling, about 20-25 minutes. Feel free to brown the top under a broiler.

11 Garnish with scallions, chives or cilantro.

Prep Time: 15 Minutes

Cook Time: 50 Minutes

Servings: 6-8

Ingredients

- 1/8 cup good olive oil
- 1/2 cup chopped pancetta or bacon –optional (feel free to leave this out, or sub vegan bacon)
- cups diced onions
- 1 cup diced carrots
- 1 cup diced fennel bulb (or sub celery)
- – 6 cloves garlic- rough chopped
- 1 teaspoon freshly ground black pepper
- 1/4 teaspoon crushed red pepper flakes, more to taste
- teaspoons salt, plus more to taste
- 2–3 medium tomatoes – diced (or a 14-ounce can diced tomatoes)
- cups lacinato kale, chopped
- Splash white wine
- cups chicken or veggie stock
- Parmesan rind (optional, but adds depth and flavor)

- cups cooked cannellini beans – or use 2 cans cannellini beans (drained, rinsed), or great northern white beans
- 1/2 cup chopped fresh Italian parsley leaves
- Grated pecorino or Parmesan – optional or try vegan parmesan
- Crusty Bread
- Rosemary Lemon Garlic Oil (for drizzling)
- ½ cup good olive oil
- zest of one large lemon
- cloves garlic, sliced
- few sprigs rosemary (or thyme, sage)

Instructions

1 Make the Lemon Garlic Rosemary Oil – place all ingredients in a small jar or bowl and let sit on the counter (or make the day before, refrigerating)

2 In a large, heavy-bottom pot or dutch oven, heat oil over medium heat. Add onions and optional pancetta and saute 6-8 minutes.

3 Lower heat to med-low and add the carrots, fennel (or celery) and garlic, salt, pepper and chili flakes, and cook another 7- 9 minutes until vegetables are tender.

4   Add the tomatoes and lacinato kale, and a splash of white wine, and continue sauteing and stirring occasionally for 7-8 minutes.

5   Add the stock and beans. Bring to soup to boil, turn heat down and simmer for 15 minutes.(You could add a Parmesan rind to the simmering soup for extra depth of flavor.)

6   Stir in fresh Italian Parsley. Adjust salt if necessary.

7   Serve in bowls with a drizzle of the flavorful lemon oil, grated Parmesan (or Romano) and crusty bread.

Prep Time: 45 Minutes

Cook Time: 15 Minutes

Servings: 8

Ingredients

Chicken skewers:

- bamboo skewers
- 1 pound chicken, (thighs or breast) sliced thin and long 1/4 inch thick x 3-4 inches long. See notes for tofu.
- 1/2 cup full fat coconut milk
- 1 tablespoon yellow curry powder or sub 1 teaspoon each- turmeric, cumin, and coriander plus 1/4 teaspoon ground ginger
- 1 tablespoon garlic, finely minced
- tablespoons brown sugar, palm sugar, agave, maple or honey
- 1/2 teaspoon salt
- teaspoons soy sauce, (or try Thai mushroom soy sauce)

- tablespoons peanut, avocado or olive oil
- 1/4 cup water

Garnishes:

- lime wedges, crushed roasted peanuts, cilantro
- Satay Sauce
- 1/3 cup peanut butter, smooth or chunky
- 1–2 tablespoons red curry paste (to taste)
- 1/3 cup full fat coconut milk
- 1 1/2 tablespoons brown sugar, palm sugar, or honey
- 1/2 teaspoon white vinegar (or lime juice)
- 1 teaspoon fish sauce
- 1/4 cup water
- Serve with Asian Cucumber Salad and Coconut Rice to create a meal.

Instructions

Chicken Satay

1. Soak 8 wooden skewers for 30-60 mins.
2. Make the marinade: mix all the marinating ingredients together in a shallow pan. Whisk together until all the ingredients are well blended.

3   Add the chicken or tofu to the marinade, and make sure both sides are covered with the sauce. Cover the meat, marinating in the refrigerator for 30 minutes or overnight, stirring occasionally. The longer it marinates, the more flavor.

4   Preheat grill to med-high. Thread all the chicken on the skewers. Don't throw away the leftover sauce- we will use it to baste the skewers on the grill.

5   Grill the chicken satay on medium-high heat at 3-4 minutes per side. Generously brush the leftover sauce on each side each time you flip the chicken over. Keep a close watch to avoid burning or overcooking the chicken as the pieces are smaller and can burn quicker, especially in the last few minutes.

6   Serve on a platter with the Satay Sauce, lime wedges, and sprinkle with crushed roasted peanuts and cilantro.

Peanut Dipping sauce:

7   Add all the ingredients to a small saucepan. Whisk until combined over medium heat letting it thicken. Taste, and adjust sweetness, salt and acid to taste. Once the sauce thickens, place it in a small bowl to serve with your chicken satay. Best served warm or at room temp.

Prep Time: 20 Minutes

Cook Time: 15 Minutes

Servings: 6

Ingredients

- pieces of skinless Salmon, about 3–4 ounces each
- teaspoons olive oil
- 2– 2 1/2 tablespoons Cajun Seasoning (or use store-bought)
- teaspoons high heat oil- avocado, coconut, ghee, more as needed.
- Buns (try these Quick Sourdough Buns), Brioche buns or any soft bun will work here!
- Dilly Ranch Dressing, Creamy Herby Hemp Dressing (or use store-bought Creamy Ranch)
- Lettuce, spinach and sprouts
- Red onion, sliced thin (or sub pickled red onions)
- Cucumber, sliced thin
- Cajun Spice Seasoning
- teaspoons smoked paprika
- teaspoons garlic powder

- teaspoons onion powder

- 1 teaspoon salt

- 1 teaspoon dried oregano

- 1 teaspoon dried thyme

- 1/2 teaspoon pepper

- 1/4–1/2 teaspoon cayenne pepper

Instructions

1. Let salmon sit at room temperature for about 20 minutes. This wills help the fish cook evenly.

2. Make the Cajun Seasoning, stirring to combine.

3. Make the Dilly Ranch Dressing(or use store-bought ranch)

4. Blacken the Salmon: Start heating a pan (cast iron or carbon steel work great) to medium-high. Meanwhile, pat the salmon dry and lightly coat with olive oil. Sprinkle cajun seasoning onto the filet, coating thoroughly about 2 teaspoons per piece. Press the spice into the fish to help it adhere. To the warmed pan add 1-2 teaspoons of high heat oil, avocado oil is great. Immediately place salmon on the pan, seasoning side down. Leave it alone, no fiddling! About 4 minutes, flip over and cook for another 3-6

minutes. This wills depend on the thickness of your filets.

5   Assemble your sandwich: Toss your greens in a bowl with dressing. Toast the bun. Layer on salmon, cucumber, onion and greens. Serve with extra dressing on the side.

Prep Time: 50 Minutes

Cook Time: 1hrs 15 Minutes

Servings: 4

Ingredients

- 1 head cauliflower – cut into 1-inch bite-size pieces
- tablespoons avocado oil or olive oil
- 1/2 teaspoon sea salt
- 14 ounce can chick peas -drained and rinsed
- 16 ounces tofu -pat dry and cut into 3/4 inch cubes
- 1/2 teaspoon kosher salt
- black pepper to taste
- tablespoons coconut oil
- cloves garlic, minced
- 1 teaspoon ginger, grated or minced
- teaspoons coconut sugar, or brown sugar

Dressing:

- 1 tablespoon apple cider vinegar
- tablespoons olive oil or avocado oil
- tablespoons madras curry powder

- 1/4 teaspoon sea salt

Garnish:

- 1/4 cup cilantro, chopped
- 1/4 cup green onions, minced
- 1 small apple, diced (optional)
- toasted cashews (optional)
- more salt to taste
- Serve with Fluffy Basmati Rice and Cilantro Mint Chutney (both optional)

Instructions

1 Preheat the oven to 425 F

2 Roast cauliflower: Cut cauliflower into bite-sized pieces and toss in a bowl with oil, salt and pepper. Spread out on a pan and roast in the oven on a baking sheet for 15-20 minutes until the pieces begin to turn golden. Remove from oven. Scoot the cauliflower over to one side of the pan and place drained chickpeas on the other side. Place back in the oven for another 5 minutes to warm the chickpeas.

3 Pan Sear tofu: Lightly blot tofu with paper towels, pressing down gently to release excess moisture. Cut

into bite-sized cubes. Heat coconut oil in a skillet over medium-high heat. Add a generous sprinkling of sea salt (about 1/2 teaspoon) and a sprinkle of pepper to the oil.

4   Add tofu to the pan, (be careful- it may pop and spit oil). Leave tofu for 3-5 minutes, once it forms a crust, flip. After 2 minutes of cooking on the second side add ginger, garlic and coconut sugar sauté for 1-2 minutes more until tofu is coated and golden. Remove from heat.

5   Mix the dressing: Add oil, apple cider vinegar, Madras Curry Powder and sea salt together in a small bowl. It will be thick, almost paste-like.

6   Combine: Gently mix the chickpeas, roasted cauliflower, caramelized tofu, and dressing in a large bowl. Toss in cilantro, scallions and apple (if using) and toss. Taste for salt and pepper.

7   Serve warm (or at room temperature) for optimum flavor over the optional basmati rice, with a spoonfull of Cilantro Mint chutney (also optional).

8   Leftovers are delicious added to salads.